THE REAL
Hoodia
Weight Loss Secrets

Jammie Morrison

TABLE OF CONTENTS

Contents

The Battle of the Bulge

To historians, the Battle of the Bulge refers to a German offensive that was launched during World War II as their troops surged through the forested regions of Belgium, France and Luxembourg during December of 1944 through January of 1945.

For most people today, however, the battle of the bulge refers to the struggle to lose weight and to keep it off as well. And to many, it can feel like an actual war! Some may say that trying to control their eating and getting some regular exercise is more difficult than giving up cigarettes or forcing oneself to go to the dentist!

What about you; are you struggling with weight? How difficult is it? Many people find that they can lose a few pounds but that they gain it right back after a few weeks or months. Some also find that as they get older they tend to gain weight no matter what they do and it gets harder to take that weight off as the years go by.

Some too come from families where just about everyone is or was overweight and they assume that weight problems are just in their genes and that there's little if anything they can do. And of course the longer you're overweight, the more you just get accustomed to it and assume that your body will just always be that way.

Just how common is it for people to struggle with their weight loss and with maintaining their weight? If you're overweight yourself you might think you're all on your own with this struggle, but let's look at some numbers and statistics about this problem.

Statistics About Weight

You may have heard the statistics that some 60% of adults in North American are overweight or obese; this problem is spreading to many other parts of the world as well. Even in places where body weight and obesity were never problems before, there are more and more cases being reported of weight problems especially as diets change and technology makes it easier to maintain a certain lifestyle.

As an example, Australian Aborigines have been reported to develop high prevalence rates of obesity, hypertension, and type 2 diabetes after transitioning to a Western lifestyle from their traditional "hunter-gatherer" lifestyle (high physical activity and low-calorie, low-fat, high fiber diet). In other words, as soon as they started following a very poor diet and no longer needed to work so hard to gather their food, they began to gain weight.

This same type of problem has happened with other cultures as well, including those in Asia, Africa, and other areas of the world. Once the "western" diet of fatty meats and cheeses, sugary foods, and heavy oils and creams were introduced, the majority of the population would gain weight. And as technology makes physical labor somewhat obsolete, this too has contributed to the problem.

Between 1976 and 2004, the prevalence of obesity (including the obese and the severely or morbidly obese) among adults aged 20-74 increased from less than 15.0% to over 35%.[1] These numbers are not decreasing these days by any means. Considered the percentages of adults that are overweight, obese, and severely obese:

	Overweight	Obese	Severely Obese	Total
1999-2000	34.0%	25.8%	4.7%	64.5%
1988-1994	33.0%	20.1%	2.9%	56.0%
1976-1980	30.6%	14.4%	No Data	46.0%

[1] CDC, National Center for Health Statistics, National Health and Nutrition Examination Survey. Health, United States, 2002. Flegal et. al. JAMA. 2002;288:1723-7. NIH, National Heart, Lung, and Blood Institute, Clinical Guidelines on the Identification, Evaluation and Treatment of Overweight and Obesity in Adults, 1998.

Notice that before 1980, doctors did not even have a classification for "severely obese" since there were not enough adults that fell into this category to record them, however, after 1999 the number of those who so overweight that they could be considered severely obese had grown to almost 5% - that's almost one in every 20 people!

So if you're overweight you're certainly not alone. It would seem that being in good shape and having one's weight under control is the oddity today, not the norm.

Health Concerns

This doesn't mean that weight problems should be ignored. Being overweight and obese is not just a problem of how you look but is a serious health risk as well. Consider the many different health problems associated with excess body weight:

- Asthma

- Arthritis

    o Obesity is associated with the development of osteoarthritis of the hand, hip, back and especially the knee.

- At a Body Mass Index (BMI) of greater than 25, the incidence of osteoarthritis has been shown to steadily increase.

- Modest weight loss of 10 to 15 pounds is likely to relieve symptoms and delay disease progression of knee osteoarthritis.

- Birth Defects

  - Maternal obesity (BMI greater than 29) has been associated with an increased incidence of neural tube defects (NTD) in several studies, although variable results have been found in this area.

- Cancers

- Cardiovascular Disease (CVD)

  - Obesity increases CVD risk due to its effect on blood lipid levels.

  - Weight loss improves blood lipid levels by lowering triglycerides and LDL ("bad") cholesterol and increasing HDL ("good") cholesterol.

  - Weight loss of 5% to 10% can reduce total blood cholesterol.

  - Overweight and obesity increase the risk of illness and death associated with coronary heart disease.

- o Obesity is a major risk factor for heart attack, and is now recognized as such by the American Heart Association.

- Carpal Tunnel Syndrome (CTS)

- Chronic Venous Insufficiency (CVI)

- Daytime Sleepiness

- Deep Vein Thrombosis (DVT)

- Diabetes (Type 2)

  - o As many as 90% of individuals with type 2 diabetes are reported to be overweight or obese.

  - o Obesity has been found to be the largest environmental influence on the prevalence of diabetes in a population.

  - o Obesity complicates the management of type 2 diabetes by increasing insulin resistance and glucose intolerance, which makes drug treatment for type 2 diabetes less effective.

  - o A weight loss of as little as 5% can reduce high blood sugar.

- End Stage Renal Disease (ESRD)

- Gallbladder Disease

  - o Obesity is an established predictor of gallbladder disease.

- Obesity and rapid weight loss in obese persons are known risk factors for gallstones.

- Gallstones are common among overweight and obese persons. Gallstones appear in persons with obesity at a rate of 30% versus 10% in non-obese.

- Gout

- Heat Disorders

- Hypertension

    - Over 75% of hypertension cases are reported to be directly attributed to obesity.

    - Weight or BMI in association with age is the strongest indicator of blood pressure in humans.

    - The association between obesity and high blood pressure has been observed in virtually all societies, ages, ethnic groups, and in both genders.

    - The risk of developing hypertension is five to six times greater in obese adult Americans, age 20 to 45, compared to non-obese individuals of the same age.

- Impaired Immune Response

- Impaired Respiratory Function

- Obesity has been found to increase respiratory resistance, which in turn may cause breathlessness.

- Decreases in lung volume with increasing obesity have been reported.

■ Infections Following Wounds

■ Infertility

■ Liver Disease

- Excess weight is reported to be an independent risk factor for the development of alcohol related liver diseases including cirrhosis and acute hepatitis.

- Obesity is the most common factor of nonalcoholic steatohepatitis, a major cause of progressive liver disease.

■ Low Back Pain

■ Obstetric and Gynecologic Complications

■ Orthopedic Complications

- Among growing youth, bone and cartilage in the process of development are not strong enough to bear excess weight. As a result, a variety of orthopedic complications occur in children and adolescents with obesity. In young children, excess weight can lead to bowing and overgrowth of leg bones.

- o Increased weight on the growth plate of the hip can cause pain and limit range of motion. Between 30 to 50 percent of children with this condition are overweight.

- Pain

- Pancreatitis

- Psychosocial Effects & Stigma

- Sleep Apnea

  - o There is a 12 to 30-fold higher incidence of obstructive sleep apnea among morbidly obese patients compared to the general population.

  - o Among patients with obstructive sleep apnea, at least 60% to 70% are obese.

- Stroke

- Surgical Complications

- Urinary Stress Incontinence

So what part of the body isn't affected when a person is overweight? It seems as if from head to toe, being overweight and obese is very dangerous to one's health overall.

There are even many other problems associated with being overweight and obese; the reason for this is that body fat attaches itself to virtually every cell of the body and acts as a sort of toxin in all systems where it's found.

You might have your own reasons for wanting to get your weight under control and to maintain it properly, but understanding the very real complications that arise from excess body weight can be even more motivation.

Why So Difficult?

If being overweight is so very dangerous, and most people would like to control their weight, why then is it so very difficult to do? What are the common reasons that many people struggle with this issue, especially now in our time since weight problems are so much more common? Let's take a closer look at those reasons here:

- **Lack of activity.** It used to be that people had to work hard to support themselves materially. Food needed to be gathered from the fields and cooking was done by scratch. Taking care of the home meant manual labor as well; furniture was repaired by hand, rugs beaten by hand, and so on. But in today's society, we drive ourselves everywhere and buy things readily made. Jobs are spent behind a desk, working on a computer while a dishwasher washes the dishes and a microwave cooks the food. Lawnmowers and vacuum cleaners are self-propelled; most other tools used to maintain the home are powered up as well. All of this adds up to a lack of physical activity every single day.

- **Calorie-dense foods eaten too often.** People have always indulged themselves in some treats and desserts; recipes for cakes and pies and other sweets can be found in the most ancient of writings. But these treats were rare and left for special occasions. The typical diet of everyday people was usually filled with wholesome foods that included vegetables, fruits, lean meats, and so on. Today however it's not unusual for people to indulge in high calorie foods every single day - packaged sweets, pizzas, and sugary sodas are commonplace. All of this results in too many calories indulged in every single day.

- **Large portions.** Compare the portions today with the portions of several decades ago and you might be shocked. What a fast food restaurant today calls a kid's meal was a meal for an adult just a generation ago. Sugary sweets and treats were small and bite-size whereas today they're the size of virtually an entire meal. You might even realize this in your own case if you're honest and think seriously about the subject - how big are the portions on your plate and in your home? Have they grown some over the past five or ten years? These jumbo portions have resulted in jumbo weight gain for many.

- **Lack of planning and preparation.** Most people would prefer to eat healthy foods if they could but in many households, both adults work outside the home and there are many other activities and responsibilities that take a toll on their schedule. After work, children need to be picked up from daycare and by the time everyone is home for dinner, they're too hungry to prepare a meal from scratch. They may also be too tired at the end of the evening to pack a good lunch for the next day.

- **Too many other options**. Fast food restaurants can be found on just about any street corner or any major city. Add to that the fact that high-calorie, high-fat foods can be found in vending machines, at gas stations, and at convenience stores everywhere. This makes it just too easy to purchase food from any of these places rather than to take the time and effort to prepare something nutritious.

There are of course many other reasons as to why it's so difficult to lose weight and to keep it off. The body is meant to protect itself from starvation by holding onto fat as much as possible. We often crave sweet foods because these will load on that fat that's needed during times of food shortages. Unfortunately our bodies are not meant to adjust to today's times where food is readily available and where many societies have too much food rather than too little.

Food manufacturers have also realized how much cheaper it is to produce processed and packaged foods that are high in calories versus harvesting fresh, wholesome foods. Corn is very easy and cheap to grow which means corn oil is easy to obtain; many packaged and processed foods are made from corn oil products or are fried in oil to help preserve them. You may have even noticed that a bag of potato chips is often cheaper than a bag of apples. When families struggle with their budget they often need to cut back on fresh foods just so that they have enough to eat.

Fast foods also are typically cheaper than other types of foods since fast food restaurants buy meat, potatoes and oil in bulk so that they get it for much cheaper than most individuals. This means that a fast food meal can actually be cheaper than a meal someplace else, making them that much more tempting to those with limited funds.

Of course taste does come into play as well. Foods that are sugary or fried in oil are usually very tasty, and it's very easy to become virtually addicted to those tastes as well. Everyone appreciates a meal that appeals to the taste buds and when vegetables and fruits just don't offer that, it's too easy to turn to foods and meals that do.

A lack of physical activity is also a problem for many; cars drive us virtually everywhere and labor-saving devices mean that there is little physical exertion needed to perform just about any job whether at home or at work. Long days behind a desk can mean that the metabolism slows down, making a person tired and fatigued at the end of the day.

Trying to schedule some exercise can be virtually impossible for most individuals and families today since in many households, both adults work secularly so there is little time to take care of household chores and responsibilities - and then to exercise on top of that. Enticing entertainment options also keep you glued to the television or computer, including video games, hundreds of television channels, "on demand" cable shows, DVDs, and of course the internet. This means that when someone does have some free time, the idea of spending that time riding a real bike or playing a real game of baseball gets tossed aside for the idea of staying in and playing a video game instead.

All of this adds up to a lack of physical activity, on top of a diet that's very high in calories; no wonder the body fat piles on for most!

What to Do?

So is it just hopeless? Is obesity just a tidal wave headed for the U.S. and other parts of the world that we can do nothing about?

What do you think about this? Do you feel just about ready to give up in your own battle of the bulge? Have you been struggling for some time and find that you just are getting nowhere?

Or maybe you've found that you can lose a few pounds but then you almost immediately gain it all back - and even more than that? Perhaps your weight has been like that proverbial yo-yo; up and down, up and down. What to do?

Before you give up just yet, let us help! In this book, we'll:

- Help you understand just why it is that people get fat in the first place. You won't need a degree in chemistry or biology to understand this, but a little bit of knowledge as to how the body works and why people become overweight can help tremendously when it comes time to make changes.

- Explain about the many different supplements there are on the market today, including a rundown of their ingredients and how they work. We'll also discuss why some are a complete waste of money and why some are even downright dangerous!

- Talk thoroughly about Hoodia, including what it is, where it comes from, and why it's the most effective supplement you can consider.

- How to help Hoodia work by being more physically active and by eating healthier, including hints and tips for sneaking in better foods and moments of activity that you might not have been able to fit into your schedule before.

The battle of the bulge is winnable, no matter what you've heard or what you've tried in the past. You can control what you eat and you can get regular exercise, if you know a few simple tips and tricks that will allow you to do just that.

And you can get the help you need by using Hoodia, a natural supplement that controls appetite and thirst without upsetting the major systems of your body. But before we get into that subject, let's take a closer look at how the body works and why you get fat in the first place!

Understanding What Makes You Fat in the First Place

So what makes you fat?

It's easy to immediately say that it's *all* in your genes but this is a very simplistic answer. While genetics may play a part in your body's storage of fat and overall size, keep in mind that humans are genetically identical now as they were a hundred years ago or a thousand years ago and yet obesity is a modern-day epidemic, the likes of which doctors and scientists have never seen.

Additionally, simply dismissing the subject by saying that you've inherited your body can mean that you refuse to take responsibility to make changes where necessary and where possible. The last thing that anyone should do is simply toss their hands in the air and say that their body is their parents' fault so there's nothing they can do about it.

Understanding what really makes you fat is going to be a very key element to losing weight and keeping it off. Think of it as you would any other part of health maintenance - if you understand what causes acne you can avoid those things to keep your skin clear; if your doctor explains to you what is causing your knee pain you can avoid putting stress on it and injuring it further.

So don't dismiss the idea of learning about what makes you fat. Knowledge is power, and learning some basics of how the body works can help you to lose weight and keep it off - and to understand how supplements like Hoodia can help as well!

Numbers Game

Your weight is something of a numbers game that involves calories taken in versus calories burned.

A calorie, by the way, is simply a unit of measurement that refers to the amount of heat needed to raise the temperature of one gram of water by one degree Celsius. The body needs energy to survive - the heart needs energy to pump, the lungs need energy to breathe, and every movement you make no matter how small involves energy as well.

When we talk about the number of calories in different food items, this isn't an actual ingredient in that food; this is just a measurement of the energy that the food will produce in the body.

This might sound like a good thing - who doesn't need more energy? Except that we're not talking about energy that spurs you to get up and be active. We're talking about stored or potential energy. This stored energy doesn't included the *motivation* to actually use it!

And what's unfortunate about this stored or potential energy is that if you don't use it through physical activity, the body will store it as fat. The fat you have on your body is actually potential energy that was never used, or calories that were never burned.

This is where that numbers game comes into play. If you eat 2,000 calories in any given day but only burn up 1,500 calories through your physical activity for that day, you're going to have 500 unused calories that the body will store as fat.

On the other hand, if you only eat 1,200 calories in one day but use up 1,500 calories through physical activity, your body will use up that extra 300 calories it needs by tapping those fat reserves, something like how you might dip into your savings account when your checking account is a bit low to pay bills.

All of these numbers don't mean that you're going to suddenly get fat the first day you eat more calories than you burn up. Usually the body adjusts its fat storage or use over the course of a week or two, which means that you might eat too many calories one day but then a few calories too little the next day, and so on. You might notice that someone who isn't overweight and who doesn't have excess body fat may have a very large meal here and there and might wonder why they don't balloon up - it's because the rest of the time they no doubt eat moderately and have achieved a balance between the calories they ingest and the calories they burn through physical activity.

This is also why you don't immediately lose weight the first time you work out or go for a long walk. You might have one good day where you burn more calories than you ingest but you need to burn enough calories to force your body to tap those fat reserves on a consistent basis.

Calories used every day.

If you're trying to lose weight, all of this information doesn't mean that you should immediately begin some type of starvation diet. When the body notices that it's low on a few calories here and there it will dip into the fat reserves but when the calories consumed are so low that it's near starvation levels, it will actually begin to eat away at its own muscles for sustenance. It's not unusual for those who have anorexia or who suffer from other eating disorders to have problems with their heart and other muscles of the body since they are literally being eaten away due to this extreme condition.

Remember that your body needs a certain number of calories just to function. Even those that are comatose still burn calories simply by having a beating heart and functioning lungs. Every movement you make, from blinking your eyes to clearing your throat to walking around and exercising, involves energy which in turn means needed calories. Denying your body of these needed calories is not a healthy way to lose weight and actually does more damage than good in the long run.

Other Factors

You might now be wondering how factors like metabolism and fat in your foods also affect your body's weight. The idea of calories in versus calories out seems very simplistic and doesn't consider these things, so what part do they play in whether or not you're overweight and how much?

Metabolism.

Your metabolism simply refers to how efficiently your body burns calories; the higher or faster your metabolism the more calories you burn per minute and the slower your metabolism, the fewer calories you burn during the same time.

Metabolism isn't something that you're simply born with; you can raise your metabolism by exercising and being active and also by building up the amount of muscle you have. The body needs to work harder to feed and maintain muscle versus fat so the more muscle a person has, the more the body is working all the time. This is one reason why so many personal trainers encourage you to add resistance training to any workout routine - if you can build just a little bit of muscle you'll be burning more calories even when you're at rest.

Your metabolism also goes up with regular exercise. When you are physically active on a regular basis you're not just burning more calories during that time of activity but also when you're at rest. This is because the heart is still beating faster and the lungs are working harder to feed and replenish those muscles you just worked on. Any increase in physical activity means more demand on the muscles and more demand needs to be met with more replenishment, so calories are burned when the body does this work.

Metabolism can also slow due to inactivity. If you've ever felt tired after doing nothing all day, this is because your metabolism has gotten slower due to there being no demands on your muscles.

To increase your metabolism and to burn more calories every day, it's important to exercise and to add some resistance training to that exercise routine as well. This will spur your heart and lungs to work all the time and will cause you to continue to burn more calories even when at rest.

Sugar.

Are all calories created equal? Not exactly. Calories in versus calories burned may be the most important aspect of what makes you fat, but the way the body responds to certain foods can also play a large role in your eating habits.

Sugar is one of the main culprits when it comes to overeating. When sugar is ingested, the body needs to break it down so that the system does not get overwhelmed. It does this by producing insulin from the pancreas. This insulin is produced when we eat, so one of the best ways the body can force the pancreas to produce more insulin is to send out hunger signals to our brain in order to force us to eat.

You may notice that when you eat large amounts of sugar you feel full at first but then get hungry an hour or so later. This is the body's way of getting you to eat so that it can have that insulin to balance that sugar level.

Sugar too is what you call empty calories, meaning that it offers no energy in return for the calories it contains. Because of the way the body just absorbs and breaks down sugar, there is no real energy you get from it.

This is why sugar is such a danger when it comes to overeating and weight problems.

Carbohydrates.

With all our talk about calories, you may be wondering why people have been paying so much attention to carbohydrates as of late. How do they come into play?

There are two types of carbohydrates - simple carbs and complex carbs. Complex carbs come from grains that have not been processed or broken down. This might include items like wheat bread or whole-grain bread.

Simple carbs are those grains that have been broken down and processed. These are white flour products such as bread or pasta. Some vegetables such as potatoes are also considered simple carbs.

The reason that carbohydrates come into play when talking about one's weight is that simple carbs break down as sugar in the body. When you have white flour products such as pasta or white bread, you might as well be eating a sugary treat.

The carbs also trigger hunger in the body for the same reason that sugar does. The body needs insulin from the pancreas to absorb and digest that sugary product, so it's not uncommon to eat simple carbs and to continue to feel hungry, either immediately or not long after. Obviously it doesn't help in controlling one's weight if the food you're eating just makes you hungrier!

Body composition.

Your body's current composition can also play a large part in how difficult or easy it is to lose weight and to maintain a healthy body weight. When you're already carrying excessive body fat, you're more likely to stay that way versus someone that has a large amount of muscle mass. Why is this? There are a few things to consider in this regard:

- The body needs to work to maintain muscle mass. Muscles need to constantly be fed fresh blood and oxygen and this means the heart is working more in order to provide that. When the heart works more, this means the body is burning calories even at rest. So those with more muscle mass are burning more calories per minute than someone with less muscle mass, even if they weigh the same amount.

- Body fat does not need that constant work in order to be maintained. Someone that is overweight because of excess body weight is not doing much to maintain itself.

- Additionally, because the body needs to exert itself in order to move that body fat around, people that are very overweight are usually very sedentary. Think of how energetic you would be if you had to carry twenty pounds of sand around with you wherever you went - chances are you would need to sit down a lot! And yet that is what happens when you have twenty pounds of extra body weight; it's easy to feel tired and lethargic all the time.

You may have noticed that some people who are very muscular and physically fit seem to never gain any weight no matter what they eat, while others who are somewhat overweight seem to have a very difficult time losing that weight no matter what they do. Body composition does play a large part in how easy or how difficult it is to lose and maintain weight.

And of course your height does come into play as well. Someone that is six feet tall is going to have more room to carry their weight without having excess body fat, whereas someone only five feet tall has lost that extra foot of height. Obviously the shorter person will need fewer calories as their bones, muscles, and everything else take up less space than the taller person. As the body needs to work harder to move itself around when there is more of it, a taller person might even be burning more calories than the shorter person simply because there is more of him or her that needs support and that the body needs to move as well. All of these factors also come into play when talking about whether or not someone has excess body fat, even if two people ingest the same amount of calories every single day.

Physical Activity

Never underestimate the importance of physical activity when it comes to weight loss and maintenance. Many people try to follow restricted diets without worrying about the amount of physical activity they get, but this is a mistake. You can only restrict your calories so much and burning those calories is going to be just as important.

Think of your body's weight as being like a car engine. When you fill the tank with gas, you need to move the car in order to burn that gas and empty the tank. Idling your car will take forever for that gas to burn.

Your body is much the same. You can only burn so many calories when you're idle or physically inactive. It's imperative to get up and get moving in order to use up those extra calories you've eaten and to cause the body to turn to the fat reserves it needs in order to sustain that activity; this will cause you to lose the body fat you're carrying.

Most people dread the idea of physical activity and exercising, but usually this is because they see it as a chore. Aerobic classes can get old and boring very quick, as can running on a treadmill or riding an exercise bike. Not to mention the expense of a gym membership or exercise equipment!

But of course physical activity doesn't mean just exercising in a structured setting or in a gym; athletes and those that are physically active with hobbies and recreational activities are burning calories just as much as someone that is actually "exercising." You are going to burn as many calories riding a stationery bike in the gym as you are when you're riding your real bike around the neighborhood! Think of playing basketball, ice or field hockey, or just chasing your children around the home - these things all burn calories very efficiently. In a later section we'll talk about how you can easily add more activity to your day.

As difficult as it might be, physical activity is absolutely necessary in order to maintain a healthy body weight. The human body was not meant to be completely sedentary and of course with today's typical diet that is so high in calories, it's no wonder that so many have problems with obesity.

Obesity is a common problem today and no doubt one of the reasons why is because we are so sedentary, especially as compared to generations ago. In the past people needed to work hard on farms and in fields in order to gather their food and prepare it. Homes needed regular maintenance and this was done by hand. While horses were used for travel people still needed to walk many places and rarely spent an entire evening just sitting; even when it was time for rest the women would still sew or knit and the men might be carving some new furniture out of wood or polishing something that needed cleaning. That constant physical activity is why they were rarely overweight or obese; the connection between maintaining one's body weight and one's physical activity level cannot be ignored.

Other Issues

Of course there may be other reasons that cause a weight problem for many. Thyroid problems, blood sugar problems, and many other personal issues can contribute to a person being overweight. If you've been overweight for many years you may do well to talk to your doctor about your own condition and contributing factors. He or she can perform a complete physical exam and talk to you about your eating habits, family history, and even your emotional health as well. Mental and emotional afflictions like depression, post traumatic stress syndrome, and others can cause fatigue and physical pain which can make it difficult to be physically active and which can affect one's blood sugar levels as well.

However, most people if forced to be honest will admit that the biggest contributor when it comes to their weight is what they put into their mouths, and how much they eat as well. An occasional cupcake or piece of fried chicken won't make anyone overweight, but eating constantly all day certainly will. Most doctors and scientists agree that humans should eat every four hours rather than the standard "three square meals" but what they eat should be very modest. The average adult female needs only 1,200-1,500 calories every day and the average male needs only 1,500-2,000. But most people eat at least twice that number of calories every day, if not even more.

And when what you eat is loaded with fat and calories, your body has no choice but to store those extra calories as fat. Eating every four hours is fine if what you eat includes fresh fruit, a small salad, and things like these but rarely is this how people actually eat.

But cutting down on one's eating can be one of the most difficult undertakings anyone can attempt. Like cigarettes, fatty and sugary foods can be addictive and the body can experience cravings and withdrawal symptoms just as if you were trying to stop smoking.

Many turn to supplements to help them in this regard, hoping that a pill or powder can make them feel full or in any other way control their appetite. Let's take a look at what some of these common supplements are and see how they work, their common side effects, and the dangers of many of them.

How Supplements Work

There have been many diet supplements on the market in the past few years and some have worked better than others, while still more have even been pulled from the market because of health concerns and side effects.

Now that you understand the factors that go into making you gain weight you can better understand how supplements work to help you take it off. Let's take a look at the most popular supplements so that we can understand the pros and cons of each.

Natural Supplements

There are many so-called natural supplements that you can purchase at health food stores and herbal stores, and some seem to work better than others. Some are known to be downright dangerous and yet they're still sold nonetheless. Since of course you want the most "bang for your buck" you want to be sure that anything you purchase will be effective.

Here's a rundown of common supplements people use for weight loss.

Bitter orange (Citrus aurantium)

Bitter orange claims to increase the number of calories burned. Some believe that it works as an ephedra substitute because its ingredients, synephrine and octopamine, are similar to the ephedrine in ephedra. The long-term effects of this supplement are unknown and it seems to have limited positive effect on those trying it. Side effects may include high blood pressure (hypertension) and heart rhythm disturbances (arrhythmias), which can lead to heart attack, stroke and even death.

Chitosan

Chitosan is a substance that blocks the absorption of body fat. While it seems to be relatively safe, it doesn't seem to be effective for weight loss.

Additionally, it usually causes constipation, bloating, and other gastrointestinal problems; some are severe. The long-term effects are so far unknown.

Chromium

Chromium is used to reduce body fat and to build muscle. Bodybuilders and weight lifters use it most often before a workout session. It seems to be relatively safe although it can cause problems for those with blood sugar problems. The long-term effects are unknown. Chromium seems to be ineffective for actual weight loss and is not typically recommended as an appetite suppressant.

Conjugated linoleic acid (CLA)

There is little evidence that CLA actually reduced appetite or builds muscles as their advertisements claim. Most users have little success with its use. It also seems to cause diarrhea, indigestions and other gastrointestinal problems for most users.

Country mallow (heartleaf)

Heartleaf contains ephedra which of course is very dangerous. It is known to be unsafe and most experts advise that you avoid using this product altogether. Ephedra itself has been taken off the market in the U.S. although it is still sold in heartleaf form and over the internet.

Salicin and white willow

The ingredients salicin or white willow are similar to aspirin; claims are that this ingredient will increase heart rate and burn calories. However, they usually have a negative effect on the system overall especially for those with diabetic nephropathy or other kidney diseases. This can also cause unnatural stress on the heart and cardiovascular system.

Green tea

Green tea is a natural tea that is very popular in many parts of Asia. This supplement is available as a tea beverage or can be taken as a pill. It seems to slightly increase a person's ability to burn fat and sometimes may result in modest, short-term weight loss.

Green tea may provide other health benefits because it contains antioxidants, those elements that attack free radicals which damage healthy cells. However, green tea may negatively interact with some medications and the results it provides are very short-term and limited when it comes to weight loss.

Pyruvate

The bodyss metabolism of glucose produces pyruvate naturally, which is why doctors and scientists began to produce it synthetically.

Limited research has been done on pyruvate and it seems that large doses might help promote modest weight loss, but side effects may include diarrhea and upset stomach as well as other gastrointestinal diseases.

Carnitine

Carnitine is found naturally in red meat and dairy products; this substance helps the body convert fatty acids to energy.

Supplements containing L-cartinine (levocarnitine) have been advertised by some as a weight-loss aid, but most research has failed to prove these claims. Scientists are considering whether L-carnitine might benefit some patients, including people receiving hemodialysis for kidney disease and people with heart disease, hyperthyroidism, dementia, male infertility or some other conditions.

Stimulants

Many diet aids contain stimulants which may include caffeine, ginseng, or guarana. These products are meant to make a person's heart beat faster which in turn gives them a short burst of energy and causes calories to be burned quicker and more efficiently.

Side effects of stimulants include irritability, sleeplessness, high blood pressure and cardiovascular problems. Additionally, most who use these products do feel a quick rush of energy but then have this followed by a "crash," where their energy levels dip dangerously low. The calories they just burned during their burst of energy don't begin to make up for the calories they won't burn because they need to rest during this crash; in the long run they're burning fewer calories overall.

There is also some research to show that stimulants of any sort can be addictive to one extent or another. You may already realize this if you drink coffee or caffeinated sodas on a regular basis; try to go a day without either of them and you probably get a tremendous withdrawal headache!

Side Effects

It's not uncommon for people to assume that since something is sold over the counter then it must be perfectly safe. This just isn't true, especially when it comes to diet pills and herbal supplements. While some claims and some ingredients are investigated by the U.S. Food and Drug Administration (FDA), not all herbal supplements are; many will print on their labels that their claims have not been established by the FDA which allows them to sell their products regardless.

The idea of effectiveness aside, it's the side effects that you might want to be most concerned with. Wasting your money on a useless product is one thing but suffering severe side effects because of that product is of course a much more serious concern.

Common side effects that may be experienced when taking diet pills (both prescription and over-the-counter) include:

- Nervousness, restlessness, and irritability

- Rambling speech, racing thoughts

- Extreme mood swings

- Trembling of the hands or other extremities

- Increased blood pressure

- Trouble sleeping, including both the quantity of sleep and the overall quality as well

- Constipation, diarrhea, excessive gas, bloating, or stomach cramps

- Urinary tract disorders

- Nausea, vomiting

- Dry mouth

- Headache

- Heart palpitations (rapid heart rate)

In very severe or extreme cases, those who take diet pills may also experience any of the following:

- Mental disturbances such as paranoia, hallucinations, delusions, depression, mania, confusion, agitation

- Numbness, particularly occurring on only one side of the body

- Skin rash, hives or unusual bruising

- Cancer, particularly of the stomach and other gastrointestinal areas

Many prescribed diet aids are lipase inhibitors, meaning that the inhibit the breakdown of fat in the body. While this might seem like a good thing, the side effects for such common diet aids include:

- More frequent bowel movements

- Inability to hold bowel movement

- Cramping

- Oily discharge in feces

- Excessive gas and bloating

The most serious side effects.

With all these side effects we've listed so far, you may wonder what would be the worst of them. Unfortunately the most serious side effect of most diet aids and pills seems to be addiction and withdrawal symptoms when the drug is stopped; these symptoms can mimic those of any number of narcotics! Withdrawal symptoms include severe mood swings, craving of the drug, and any number of physical ailments and problems associated with withdrawal.

Prescribed Products

Most prescribed and commercial diet products are a mixture of chemicals that work on the brain's hunger signals or those that affect the production of insulin from the pancreas which also affects hunger. Some of the more dangerous ingredients simply speed up the heart rate, which will cause the body to burn calories but which will also put an unnecessary burden on the heart and which can lead to all sorts of heart diseases and conditions.

Other ingredients will cause the body to lose moisture which means you may lose some water weight, and still others cause the colon to spasm which will make your bowels move unnaturally; we call these laxatives.

Many of these chemicals and their processes are very dangerous to your overall health. They can cause long-term damage to your heart, lungs, and tissue and cells of the body. Some who abuse these types of products for long periods of time may suffer irreparable damage to their digestive system as well.

Let's take a closer look at many of these common commercial and prescribed products so that you can better understand how many artificial diet supplements work and why they may be not only ineffective but downright dangerous.

Meridia and Xenical

In the mid-1990s, doctors also prescribed the popular appetite suppressant Redux which was the combination of two chemicals calls phentermine and fenfluramine; the suppressant soon adopted the name "phen-fen."

Redux were withdrawn from the market in 1997 because it was found to cause damage to heart valves and other cardiovascular diseases. Reports of rapid heartbeats, heart attacks, and even death were associated with the use of phen-fen.

However taking phentermine alone has not been associated with these side effects of the fenfluramine-phentermine combination, so many diet aids contain phentermine alone. One such popular drug is called Meridia.

Another type of prescription weight loss drug is one that works by inhibiting the absorption of fat into the system. Xenical is one such example of this medication; it works by blocking some 30% of fat ingested from being absorbed into the body. The medication option named Alli is one form of Xenical.

Side effects with both medications.

The common side effects with Meridia and Xenical both include:

- Increased heart rate, rapid pulse
- Increased blood pressure

- Sweating

- Constipation, bloating, gas, other gastrointestinal irritations

- Insomnia, including the inability to get to sleep and to stay asleep or to get deep and restful sleep

- Excessive thirst and dry mouth

- Lightheadedness, dizziness, feeling faint especially upon standing

- Drowsiness during the day

- Stuffy nose and other sinus problems

- Headache

- Anxiety, depression, irritability, mood swings

Specific side effects with Xenical include cramping, flatulence, leakage of stool, oil in stool, increased number of bowel movements, and the inability to control bowel movements.

While these side effects are typically mild and temporary for some, they may be worsened by eating foods that are high in fat since the medication does not allow this fat to be absorbed into the system and instead it passes through the digestive system. Patients who take Xenical should eat a low-fat diet (less than 30% of calories from fat) before starting treatment and during treatment with this medication.

Because Xenical reduces the absorption of some vitamins that you normally get through dietary fat, patients taking Xenical should take a multivitamin every single day.

The medication Meridia seems to affect the cardiovascular system of those who take it. Anyone with high blood pressure, heart disease, a history of heart attack or stroke, or irregular heartbeats should avoid taking Meridia. Patients taking Meridia must have their blood pressure and heart rate monitored on a regular and consistent basis.

As with these other side effects, both Meridia and Xenical carry with it the risk of addiction and withdrawal symptoms upon stopping the medication. All prescription medications except Xenical are considered controlled substances meaning that doctors need to follow strict guidelines when prescribing them and must monitor their patient's health constantly to check for any potential side effects.

Limited effectiveness.

Many who take these drugs also seem to develop a tolerance for them, meaning that their effectiveness wears off after a certain period of time. Some find that they may lose a certain amount of weight for up to six months but after this time their weight levels off or they may even begin to gain it back even if they are continuing to take the medication. This means that they may be risking the potential side effects without the drug having any effectiveness or results for them.

Doctors even typically agree that most medications, even those strong enough to be available only by prescription, have only limited success. Controlling one's appetite and learning to make better choices as well as being physically active on a regular basis is the only real way to lose weight and keep it off.

Cost.

The cost of these medications also needs to be taken into account. Prescriptions for weight loss drugs are rarely if ever covered by one's health insurance, which means that an individual might shell out hundreds of dollars over the course of a year just to have these. And if the effectiveness of the medication wears off after about six months, what good is that? You're paying for something that is no longer effective for you.

Natural and herbal supplements for weight loss always seem to be the most recommended by experts. This is because they're not made of harsh chemicals that act as stimulants to the nervous system or digestive system. They usually don't have the side effects that prescription medications do and seem to remain effective as long as they're taken.

Hoodia is being touted today as one of the most natural and safest weight loss aids there is. Let's take a closer look at this particular substance to see why that is and why it may be the best weapon you can have in your arsenal when it comes to the battle of the bulge.

How Hoodia Helps

So why Hoodia? Why should you consider this natural herbal supplement as being a recommended option for you?

There are a few reasons why Hoodia has become one of the most popular diet aids ever discovered and packaged. A closer look at this substance and how it works on the human body can help you to understand those reasons.

What is Hoodia

Notice Wikipedia's explanation of Hoodia:

"Hoodia is a genus of 13 species in the flowering plant family Apocynaceae, under the subfamily Asclepiadoideae. They are stem succulents, described as 'cactiform' because of their remarkable similarity to the unrelated cactus family. They can reach up to 1m high and have large flowers, often with flesh color and strong smell.

Many Hoodia species are protected plants, typical of the Namib Desert, ranging from Central Namibia to southern Angola, especially in plains and rocky areas. Common names include 'Bushman's Hat' and 'Queen of the Namib'.

Several species are grown as garden plants, and one species, Hoodia gordonii, is being investigated for use as an appetite suppressant.

On January 18, 2008, the Botanic Gardens Conservation International (representing botanic gardens in 120 countries) stated that '400 medicinal plants are at risk of extinction, from over-collection and deforestation, threatening the discovery of future cures for disease.' These included Yew trees (the bark was used for cancer drugs, paclitaxel, although current licensed syntheses do not); Hoodia (from Namibia, source of weight loss drugs); half of Magnolias (used as Chinese medicine for 5,000 years to fight cancer, dementia and heart disease); and Autumn crocus (for gout). The group was said to have found that five billion people rely upon traditional plant-based medicine for health care."

You will notice that even Wikipedia, which in no way is associated with the sales of Hoodia, claims that it is being investigated for use as a weight loss drug. As the site also points out, people have been using plant-based medicines for health care for centuries.

Let's examine how Hoodia works in the system once it's ingested so that we can better understand how it can help with weight loss and maintenance.

History of Hoodia

Many populations in Southern Africa have been using plants including Hoodia for problems like indigestion and infections for many centuries. Hoodia came to the attention of westerners however when it was learned that they would also use the meat of the plant to suppress their appetite and thirst during long hunting trips in the Kalahari Desert.

Again quoting Wikipedia, "In 1977, the South African Council for Scientific and Industrial Research (CSIR) isolated the ingredient in hoodia—now known as P57—which is responsible for its appetite-suppressant effect, and patented it in 1996.

The CSIR collaborated with the pharmaceutical company Pfizer to isolate active ingredients from the extracts and look into synthesizing them for use as an appetite suppressant."

P57 likely has an effect on the brain's hypothalamus, which helps regulate appetite. In other words, Hoodia tricks your brain into thinking you're full even if your stomach technically isn't. By blocking hunger pains and sending out that "full" signal, you're less likely to eat when you don't need any more food.

Much like protein.

This "full" signal to the brain making it feel full is not limited simply to the Hoodia plant. Protein of all sorts also have a chemical in them that makes the brain think the body is full. This is why many people have more success with weight loss when they add more protein to their diet - they feel full faster than when they're eating carbohydrates or sugars, which don't contain these chemicals. Think about this for a moment - you can eat and eat and eat all sorts of sugary foods and you may feel nauseated but not full. On the other hand a nice steak or helping of chicken is going to make you feel sated very quickly.

Remember that everything that happens in the body is controlled by the brain and the nerve signals that it receives and translates. You don't actually hear with your ears, but the ears receive sound waves which trigger the nerves in your ears to send those signals to the brain so that it translates that signal as sound. This is true of all the senses and many other bodily functions as well. The heart beats because the brains tells it to do just that, and we eat because the stomach sends a signal to the brain stating that it needs more food - so in turn the brain makes us feel those hunger pangs.

Sending the wrong signals to the brain is one reason why many people overeat. They eat out of boredom or because they're nervous or tense. Think of how this might be true in your case. Do you sometimes feel hungry when you know you're just bored, nervous, upset, lonely, irritated, or for some reason other than actually needing food? That's because the brain is receiving the wrong signals and sending out the wrong impulses, spurring one to eat when hunger is not an issue.

If we can send the right signals to the brain and tell it that we're full, imagine how much food could be avoided! The body only needs so much food to exist and to be healthy and yet often we just eat and eat and eat, thinking that we're hungry when we're really not. But if those hunger pangs could be stopped in the brain where they originate, we would save literally hundreds of calories every day!

But does Hoodia work? And what are the side effects, if any? Let's take a look at this next.

Does it Work

Mark Blumenthal, the founder and executive director of the American Botanical Council, a nonprofit research organization in Austin, Texas, seems to think so. Citing a laboratory study about the effectiveness of Hoodia, Blumenthal stated: "We can only say the evidence available to us right now, which is considered inadequate, suggests that there is some type of appetite-suppressing mechanism in some of the naturally occurring chemicals in Hoodia."

The "inadequate" evidence he was citing was produced by Doctor David MacLean, an adjunct associate professor of Brown University in Providence, Rhode Island, and a former researcher for Pfizer; this evidence was reported in a study that Doctor MacLean conducted on the P57 molecule in Hoodia. Doctor MacLean's study reported that P57 did affect the brain's hypothalamus, which controls and regulates appetite.

Another study was conducted around the same time by Doctor Richard M. Goldfarb, director of Bucks County Clinical Research, an organization that conducts studies for pharmaceutical and other companies. Doctor Goldfarb administered Hoodia to seven test subjects who were told to take two Hoodia tablets a day, eat a balanced breakfast and take a multivitamin, but not to change their eating and exercise habits.

In this particular study the starting weights of the participants ranged from 193 to 345 pounds and they lost, on average, 3.3% of their body weight. The median loss over the 28-day study was 10 pounds, and the participants also reported that they wound up eating about half of what they had eaten before!

Doctor Goldfarb's report stated, "Hoodia works within the satiety center of the brain by releasing a chemical compound similar to glucose but up to 100 times stronger. The hypothalamus receives this signal as an indication that enough food has been consumed and this in turn decreases the appetite."[2]

Yet another study was conducted by Phytopharm, a U.K. based company that states that their participants noted a reduction in average daily calorie intake by about 1,000 a day after only two weeks of using Hoodia. Their participants also noted a decrease in appetite and body fat as well.

---

[2] As quoted on WebMD.com.

Just about every study group and research facility that has studied Hoodia has reported that it has some measure of success for everyone that uses it. While it doesn't mean that suddenly everyone that uses it will suddenly start eating like a bird, it does mean that it can help to reduce calories every single day. And of course just a few calories reduced every day can really add up - imagine cutting out even 100 calories every single day; that's 3000 calories each month! By doing nothing else you could then lose a pound a month with even this slight change; that's 12 pounds or one dress size every single year.

But what about endorsements for Hoodia? Has anyone not associated with the diet industry ever said anything positive about this plant? Or is it all just hype?

Endorsements

It's difficult to just take any endorsements of any product at face value. Celebrities and others are paid to say what they do on a commercial and many don't care about whether or not what they're saying is true.

And of course even if something did work on one person this doesn't guarantee that it will work on someone else. Everyone's system is different and everyone has different struggles when it comes to weight loss and maintenance.

But that doesn't mean that Hoodia has been ignored completely by the mainstream media. Most who endorse Hoodia as an appetite suppressant note how Leslie Stahl, a "60 Minutes" reporter and correspondent, traveled to the Kalahari Desert to sample the Hoodia gordonii plant and to report on its supposed suppressant qualities.

Ms. Stahl, during the report, ate a small piece of the plant herself and then said that after eating it she did notice a marked decrease in her appetite for the entire day, stating that she wasn't hungry at all for the rest of the day.

This isn't to say that Leslie Stahl actually endorses Hoodia per se but note that her job as a reporter and correspondence would cause her to report the plant's effectiveness, or ineffectiveness, honestly and fairly. If she had felt no change in her system she no doubt would have noted that for her story.

There probably isn't a fairer correspondent and reporter than Leslie Stahl and while her story cannot be taken as an actual endorsement for the use of Hoodia, the fact that she would report it having appetite suppressant qualities should give anyone pause for consideration.

Side Effects

What about side effects? This is very important to consider because of course it doesn't matter if something works to help you lose weight if it harms your health or any part of your body in the process.

Doctor Mark Blumenthal, mentioned in one of the studies above, stated that he had not received any consumer reports of safety problems with Hoodia. Doctor Goldfarb, whose participants reported decreased appetite up to half of what they had before, also stated his participants reported none of the jitteriness and insomnia that many diet pill patients report.

Consider the typical side effects of most diet pills and aids. Even the ones that are prescribed by the doctor carry with them some pretty unpleasant conditions - loose stools that you can't control, nausea, flatulence, and dizziness. It would also seem preferable to stay overweight than to deal with those things on a daily basis!

As a matter of fact, there seems to be a real lack of reports of side effects of Hoodia no matter who tries it and who is doing the research. This is one reason why so many prefer this supplement over other, harsher supplements.

Precautions

This of course doesn't mean that Hoodia should just be taken at will and without any regard or thought for potential side effects. Anything taken through the digestive system is going to be filtered through the liver and a buildup of the supplement is possible if you take too much. Additionally, everyone system is different and everyone is sensitive to different things. It's imperative that if you are going to take Hoodia in any amount that you pay attention to any potential side effects that you may suffer. Be especially attentive to:

- Insomnia or disturbed sleep of any type.

- Nervousness, irritability, mood swings.

- Increased heart rate or heart palpitations.

- Rashes or hives.

- Dry mouth.

- Headaches.

- Lightheadedness, dizziness, or fainting spells.

- Difficulty breathing.

- Nausea and vomiting.

- Trembling hands.

Any of these symptoms can signal an allergic reaction to the ingredients in Hoodia. If you experience any of these it's important to stop taking Hoodia and to see your doctor.

You also need to talk to your doctor about taking Hoodia if you're taking any other medications as herbal supplements can interfere with their effectiveness. And because it gets filtered through the liver you shouldn't take Hoodia if you have liver diseases or conditions.

It's also not recommended that pregnant or nursing women take Hoodia because it's simply not known how it would affect the pregnancy or the nursing child.

Hoodia suppresses not only the appetite but thirst as well. It's important that you keep yourself hydrated when taking Hoodia so be sure that you drink plenty of water and other fluids even if you're not necessarily thirsty. Extra hydration is necessary when you're trying to lose weight anyway, so be sure you have at least eight glasses or two liters of water every single day.

What to Avoid

As with anything else you might take by way of medication or supplement, there are some things you want to avoid when using Hoodia. Consider the following:

- Do not take too much or double up on your doses. Every package will tell you the recommended dosage and you should follow that carefully.

- Avoid excessive caffeine when using Hoodia. This is because caffeine is a diuretic, meaning that it causes you to lose water in your system. Since Hoodia may suppress your natural thirst, it's easy to become dehydrated when you combine Hoodia with excessive caffeine. Switch to decaffeinated coffee and sodas.

- Don't use other diet aids and appetite suppressants while using Hoodia. Too much of any suppressant can cause these elements to build up in the liver and cause damage to the digestive system.

- Make sure you follow a healthy eating pattern when taking Hoodia. Remember that the body needs some amount of calories and food even when you're overweight. Starving yourself is only going to cause harm to your system.

It's also important to remember that Hoodia will not just automatically and magically melt body fat away without any effort on your part. You will still need to watch what you eat and exercise regularly. Not only will these two habits help you maintain a healthy body weight but they'll also encourage your good health as well. While having your appetite suppressed by Hoodia will help tremendously in allowing you to exercise more regularly and in weight loss, you will need to be careful of what you eat when you are hungry. Hoodia won't slap that candy bar out of your hand or make your choose some lean and healthy eggs over pancakes when it's time for breakfast!

But as we've said, exercising and eating right can be two of the most difficult endeavors anyone can try. However, with a few simple tips and tricks you might find that it's much easier to sneak in some exercise and healthier food options than you imagined. Let's take a look at that subject in the next sections.

Managing Physical Activity

If a good part of weight loss is burning off those calories that you do ingest, how can you increase your physical activity levels? After all, if it were so easy to just get up and exercise then probably everyone would do it. And while gyms are usually packed right after the first of the year when everyone makes their resolutions and tries to stick to them, it's not unusual for people to give up their workout schedule after just a few days or weeks.

Remember that no appetite suppressant in the world is going to make you stop eating completely, and this wouldn't be healthy anyway. You need to exercise regularly in order to take off the excess weight and to keep it off as well.

In this section we'll cover a few simple tips and tricks you can apply to get you up and moving.

Don't Exercise

If you want to be physically active and therefore burn more calories, why do we say that you shouldn't exercise?

Probably one of the reasons that many people abandon their workout routines is because it's so incredibly boring to be on a treadmill or elliptical machine time and time again. Even an aerobics class can get very tedious.

So rather than do any of these things over and over again, pick some physical activities that you enjoy that are going to get you up and active and which will serve as your workout routine. Remember that vigorous activity is going to burn calories whether that activity is in a stuffy and boring gym or outside in the fresh air.

Consider any of the following activities that you might enjoy:

- Bike riding with the kids.

- Walking the dogs.

- Playing baseball or softball.

- Bowling.

- Dancing with a spouse or partner, or taking a dance class.

- Playing hockey.

- Golfing.

- Swimming.

- Skiing or snowboarding.

- Playing tennis.

Notice that none of these activity ideas are very difficult and if done for fun, they don't involve heavy competition and you shouldn't need specialized lessons. And if you're doing something that you enjoy, you're more likely to keep up with it as time goes on.

We often forget that doing something we love can count as exercising, if it's active enough to actually get the heart rate going and to put some demands on the muscles. You can even challenge yourself in many ways by taking your activity levels one step further - walk around the golf course rather than get a cart, or try line dancing or salsa dancing rather than slow dancing. Keep up a brisk pace when walking the dogs rather than lagging behind and challenge yourself to some fast-paced laps when swimming; these things can really help to burn those calories and to keep the weight under control. But in any case, don't think of it as exercise and you'll be more likely to keep up with it.

Keep a Record

How often have you thought to yourself that it was just yesterday that you did something, and then you realized that it has actually been many days or weeks since you did? You might think that it's only been a day since you went to the supermarket and yet it was really a week ago, or that you just called your mother on the phone the day before yesterday when it was really a few weeks ago.

So it is with exercise. You may think that you're being active four or five times during the week but in truth you work out maybe once or twice. You think you were on the treadmill just yesterday but it was really three days ago. When you keep a record you see how much time you're really spending being active, or not. This can be great motivation to stay on a regular schedule.

You can also keep track of how much exercise or activity you're getting as well as how often. When you go for a walk, keep track of the time and mark how long you're out. The same with just about any other exercise or activity. Again, it's easy to assume you're walking around the neighborhood for an hour but it's really just 30 minutes, or that you were dancing for three hours when it was just one hour. When you see your numbers right there in black and white, you can realize where you might need to make some adjustments to really challenge yourself and to make sure your activity is actually accomplishing something.

Ask for Help

It can be difficult to talk to a family member or friend about your need for more exercise but sometimes when you do, you find out that he or she is in the same situation! And very often they're happy to help.

This doesn't mean that he or she will be following you in their car while you jog down the sidewalk like a scene from a "Rocky" movie, but it does mean that you can work together to get active and stay active.

A friend or family member can help to brainstorm ideas on things you can do together, or they may know of something that has helped them such as a certain workout routine or tape. When you have someone that is expecting you to show up for an exercise class or to go swimming with or with whom you can join a bowling or baseball league, this can mean that you're less likely to neglect your plans.

It's often helpful to be with someone when you do go to an exercise class or when you want to go for a walk. Having a good friend that you can talk to about your class or talk with while walking, or not feeling as if you're walking into your gym alone, can be a very reassuring factor. You can also go dancing together and not feel as if you'll be hit on by strangers!

Talking over your new plans and need for exercise can be a great thing to do if you have a friend or family member that would be understanding. If not, think about how you can get something together with coworkers or neighbors. Have you met nearby families through your child's school with whom you're friendly? Or what about those at your church or religious organization? Or do you engage in volunteer work so that you've met someone that might want to go walking a few times per week? If you brainstorm about your possibilities you might be surprised at the people that are available and that may be looking to get active again as well.

Start Slow and Stretch

If you haven't been physically active in some time or if you're very overweight, it's going to be important that you start slow and make sure you stretch your body before and after exercising. There are a few important reasons for this. One, when you're overweight you are putting added pressure on the joints and ligaments already. Being active puts that much more pressure on them and there is increased risk of injury if you're overly active all at once. Slamming onto the pavement to jog or play tennis also means slamming onto your joints, including your ankles, knees, and hips. You're also putting that much more pressure on your heart and lungs to make them work harder to support your physical activity. If you haven't been very active your heart probably isn't very strong so it needs to build up that strength gradually.

Stretching is also important because if you've been physically inactive your muscles are probably tense and stiff. This is due to the lack of blood circulation you experience when inactive. A gentle stretching routine when done on a regular basis can increase blood flow to your muscles and loosen them up as well as strengthen them. This also prepares those muscles for the demands you'll be making on them when you exercise.

You might dismiss routines such as tai chi or yoga but these gentle stretching routines can do a world of good. You don't need to believe in the spiritual aspects of either to follow the simple stretching and deep breathing instructions that such routines offer, and if you do them regularly you will probably find that your entire body feels loose and limber and that your breathing is improved as well.

If you're very overweight or have any other physical considerations you may want to visit your doctor before beginning an exercise routine. He or she can advise you on what types of exercises are best for you and may also point out any that should be avoided as well.

Consider the Benefits

Sure, you can lose weight with exercise but this isn't the only benefit derived from regular physical activity. If you seriously consider the benefits of exercise you may be more motivated to continue with it even when you're bored or tempted to give up. Reminding yourself of the good that you're doing to your entire body can help you when you are exercising as you keep in mind how you're helping yourself in both small and large ways.

Consider the many benefits of regular exercise and physical activity:

- Reducing the risk of cardiovascular disease as well as strengthening the heart muscles.

- Improving ability to manage blood sugar levels which in turn can ward off or help to control diabetes, hyperglycemia, and hypoglycemia.

- Reducing and controlling high blood pressure.

- Easing chronic and acute pain in all joints and muscle groups.

- Reducing the risk of many cancers; this is especially true when body weight is controlled as obesity is often associated with many types of cancer.

- Improving emotional and mental health disorders such as depression and producing an uplifted mood, as well as assisting with stress.

- Preventing osteoporosis.

- Strengthening the bones.

- Improving digestion and helping with gastrointestinal disorders.

- Improving sleep quantity and quality.

- Reducing levels of the "bad" LDL cholesterol while increasing levels of "good" HDL cholesterol.

- Reducing the buildup of plaque on the arteries and reversing the process of the hardening of the arteries.

- Strengthening the lungs and improving breathing.

- Improving posture which can cut down on lower and upper back pain and other stresses on joints and tendons in the legs and ankles.

Regular exercises is also associated with longevity; while there is still much research to be done in this regard, it is true that a stronger heart and a stronger set of lungs can help to keep you healthier in many ways and therefore avoid many conditions that can claim your life far too early.

Get the Kids Involved

How many times have you tried to get out of doing something you knew you should do only to have the kids give you a hard time about it? Kids can work well in keeping you active if you decide to keep them involved in your exercise routine. They're also typically more naturally active than adults so they may want to get outside and be active even when the grownups don't.

A good thing you can do to keep the kids involved is to have them come up with ideas on what the family can do to stay active. Ask them what they would like to do on a Saturday afternoon whether it's tossing around a baseball or going to the park.

You can also have the kids work with you to come up with a chart or calendar to keep you active on a regular basis. Have them make notes as to how much everyone exercised and for how long. It can become a coloring project for them - choose different colors when you increase your exercise or have a particularly strenuous day. You can dress it up with stickers and other decorations and they'll love exercising all the more.

Obesity is a problem for children as well as adults these days so getting them active now can help to set a good example that they'll hopefully follow for the rest of their lives. Think of this as an investment in their future health as well as for yours.

Remember that Hoodia will help to control your appetite but you can only restrict your eating so much; physical activity will help to burn the extra calories you do have every day and will force your body to start using up those fat reserves as well. So help Hoodia do the job it's meant to do by getting active every single day! You'll not only look better but you'll be healthier overall as well.

Eating Better

Eating better is a challenge for anyone. As with exercise, if you could just eat healthy all the time without a problem or challenge, everyone would be doing it. Recognizing and overcoming those challenges is overwhelming for many, and while Hoodia will do much to help with controlling your appetite so that you don't overeat, this doesn't mean that you won't give in to the occasional temptation of a sugary or fatty snack that will undo all the good Hoodia will do for you.

There are some quick and easy changes you might consider when it comes to your own diet that will ensure the maximum benefit from Hoodia and to encourage your best health as well. Let's take a look at them in this section.

Watching Calories

Why is it so hard to keep track of calories consumed and to make sure you eat only a modest amount every day? Probably one of those reasons is that there are many foods that are calorie-dense, meaning they have a lot of calories packed into their small size. It's possible that you're not eating a lot of food but you are consuming a lot of calories.

As an obvious example of this, consider a typical breakfast for many people. Two medium eggs are 140 calories, whereas a cup of most raisin bran cereals have around 200 calories, not counting the milk you pour on top. So a breakfast of approximately can mean literally hundreds of extra calories.

Think of how many food items you consume that pack a lot of calories into a very small package. Start with breakfast foods - toaster pastries, pancakes, waffles, and cereal are all typically very high in sugar and calories for the small amount of food you actually get. Bread too is another culprit, so toast or muffins can also be very calorie-dense.

Let's move on to lunch. Fast food items typically are known for their high calorie count; fries are often the worst but of course many moderate hamburgers can have about half of the calories you're supposed to get all day even before you add things like mayonnaise, bacon, cheese, and so on. A large deli sandwich can be just as high in calories if you count the bread, meat, cheese, mayo, and all the extras.

There are many foods that people eat today on a regular basis that are very high in calories for the small amount of food you actually get. Sugary desserts and treats are of course the worst; a small cupcake can be as much as 200 calories for the little wad of food you're getting! Eating these types of calorie-dense foods on a regular basis can be a surefire way to pack on the pounds quickly and easily.

Fewer calorie-dense foods.

You can't just cut out the calorie-dense foods you eat; you need to replace them with something else or you'll go hungry. So consider some less calorie-dense foods you can eat instead of those sugary and so-called "empty" foods:

- Protein usually has fewer calories per ounce than most other foods; lean chicken or pork has fewer calories than potatoes or bread, as will eggs. Try to eat lean protein as much as possible, such as eggs for breakfast and chicken for lunch rather than potato soup.

- Most vegetables are also less calorie-dense. Leafy vegetables such as varieties of lettuce are good but so are beans, cauliflower, broccoli, and so on. Incorporate these into as many meals as you can to help fill you up without loading on those extra calories.

- If you must have something sweet, opt for fresh fruit rather than packaged snacks.

- Wheat or whole-grain bread typically has fewer calories than white bread. With most breads, the darker it is the fewer calories it will have. Be sure to read the package for exact calorie counts.

- Make small changes when it comes to canned or bottled food items. Switch to reduced calorie salad dressing and mayonnaise. Have soup made with a broth base rather than creamy styles.

Track Calories

Most support groups for weight loss encourage and instruct their members to track what they eat throughout the day so that you know how your calorie intake is progressing. Many people who keep an accurate track are actually shocked at what they're eating and how quickly those calories add up!

You might think it's difficult to track your calories but today you can find calorie listings for virtually any food and restaurant online. Most people eat the same foods over and over again and have the same meals at restaurants when they do eat out, so you can find your listings in advance of eating and then check calorie amounts for anything else you eat.

Here are some good websites to help you track calories:

- http://caloriecount.about.com/

- http://www.calorieking.com/

- http://www.weightlossforall.com/calorie-content-of-foods.htm

- http://www.caloriecountercharts.com/chart1a.htm

- http://www.peertrainer.com/dfcaloriecountera.aspx

- http://calorielab.com/index.html

Keeping a record of your calories shouldn't be that difficult either. You can purchase a monthly calendar or simply make up a grid that represents your week or month and write in your total calories every day. If you keep this calendar or grid out and in front of you, such as clipping it to the refrigerator, you're much less likely to cheat on your calorie count since you can see how well you did or didn't do for the past few days.

Healthier Foods

If you're going to watch your calories you might immediately begin seeing how quickly those calories add up. You might also be surprised at how often you eat foods that just aren't healthy for you - fast foods, fried foods, sugary treats, and things like this are common for many.

So if you want to cut down on those types of foods, how can you choose healthier foods as a substitute? Here are some things to remember.

What is healthy for you?

Probably one of the reasons that people have a hard time choosing healthier foods is because they often don't know what healthy foods actually are. Many people today rely on packaged foods or sugary cereals for breakfast, fast food for lunch, and frozen meals or fried foods for dinner. If you've grown up this way it may be difficult to understand how unhealthy these foods are and to not just choose but prepare healthier options.

Here are some suggestions for what is healthier for you:

- Fruits and vegetables of course are always the healthiest choices you can make. While fresh is best, frozen is good. You can also steam them for a side dish.

- Lean meats such as chicken, turkey, lean pork or fish are healthier than fatty meats such as beef. Processed meats like hot dogs or canned meats are usually the fattiest.

- Packaged foods are usually processed so much that they have little nutritional content left. Many foods are also fried in oil as a preservative. Pastries and cakes of any sort are usually very high in oil and sugar.

- Sugar is usually added to many canned and bottled foods in order to make them taste better. If you check the ingredients on soups, salad dressings, salsa, and things like these you'll often see sugar listed as a first ingredient. Being able to make your own items rather than having these canned items can be much healthier.

- There are very few choices you can make at fast food restaurants that can be considered healthy. Even salads can pack on the calories once you add bacon, cheese, and salad dressings. It's always recommended that you avoid fast food meals just as much as possible.

- Food preparation also will contribute to whether or not food is health. Frying anything is going to make it unhealthy. Adding heavy creams, cheese, mayonnaise, and items like these also packs on the calories.

Think of how all these better choices might come into play in your case and think about where some changes can be made. If you're not sure about how to make changes, let's talk about some options for you.

Sneaking in healthy foods.

Switching to healthier foods doesn't need to be as difficult as you might think it would be. Sometimes just being sneaky can go a long way toward helping you to eat better and to make healthier choices. Here are some things to think about.

- **Plan ahead.** Many fast food meals are eaten because everyone is hungry and no one has planned meals or grocery shopping. If you plan ahead for what you'll need to prepare for breakfast, lunch, dinner, and snacks for the week and are sure to do some shopping, you'll be more likely to have what you need. It shouldn't take that long to make a shopping list; just check what you already have versus what you need as you make a meal plan for the week.

- **Have a vegetable or fiber with every meal.** For breakfast, make an omelet with spinach, onions and peppers. Or be sure to have some whole grain or whole wheat toast. Have a side salad with every dinner and load up on the steamed vegetables as side dishes. Forego your white flour rolls for whole wheat.

- **Substitute chicken or pork where possible.** For instance, when making chili leave out the beef and use chicken. Have a grilled chicken sandwich rather than a hamburger. Make chicken stew instead of beef stew. If you can substitute one of these leaner meats for the fattier cuts of beef you're still satisfying your cravings for meat but are cutting down on that excess fat.

- **Adjust your recipes.** When making any type of dessert from scratch, cut down on the amount of sugar that you use or try a substitute like applesauce. You can also typically sneak in some wheat bran for most recipes in order to fill up on fiber. Don't overdo it; just add a quarter cup to a cake mix or to pancakes in the morning.

- **Add lettuce and tomato.** You can usually add lettuce and tomato to sandwiches of any type, as well as to hamburgers and even hot dogs! Sprouts also bulk up a sandwich with leafy greens. And if you start to add just a thin amount you can gradually increase how much you add to your sandwiches so that soon you're eating more vegetables than you are the fatty meats and cheeses!

- **Think about your snacks.** What do you have in the afternoon when you're at the office and start to get hungry? Do you immediately grab a bag of potato chips from the vending machine? Why not bring in an apple or banana every day instead? Or you can pack some baby carrots and a small amount of reduced calorie ranch dressing for dip. At night, have low-fat popcorn rather than popcorn drenched in butter or more potato chips. Give your snacks some consideration and think of how you can use these as an opportunity to sneak in some healthy foods.

Learn to cook.

Learning to cook and to use the right tools in the kitchen cannot be overemphasized. When you use items like a rotisserie or a tabletop grill you can really cook healthier foods with less fat. And if you learn how to spice your foods and season them properly you can get away from adding butter, oil or sugar to give your food some flavor.

You might think that you already know how to cook but think seriously about the methods that you use and what you prepare. If you find yourself deep frying or pan frying most of your dishes, you can probably stand to learn a few new tricks. This doesn't mean that you need to start preparing everything from scratch or that you need to spend hours slaving over a hot stove; if you spend some time online you'll probably find plenty of recipes that are simple and that are purposely designed for the busy lifestyle. There are also many things you can do the night before so that you have a nice meal the next day, such as putting all your ingredients into a slow cooker and putting it into the refrigerator; the next morning you simply plug it in and let it cook.

There are many spice blends and seasoning mixes available to you at the supermarket if you're still unsure of your abilities. Most of these have cooking instructions printed right on the back. If you want to make some simple chili or stew or soup or even a rotisserie chicken you can use these seasoning blends to spice things up and chances are you won't even miss all the fat and oil and sugar you once used.

Groups and Meal Plans

What about eating support groups or prepackaged meal plans? Will these work for you?

Whether or not to consider any of these options is going to be up to you. There are some groups that seem to have a lot of success with their members while others still struggle with weight even after attending their meetings for months and years. Packaged meals can be a good way to plan your eating - if you can control yourself and not eat everything all at once!

There is the cost of these things as well. Most support groups charge a weekly fee for every single meeting while some are nonprofit and may only ask for contributions. Packaged meals can cost half over again the meals if you had made them from scratch; some are even double the cost. Only you know your budget.

Here are some things to consider:

- What about your level of commitment? If you join a support group you may need to show up every week for months and even years. How will that fit into your schedule and will you stick with this?

- Will prepackaged meals give you the vitamins and minerals you need? Many don't have fresh vegetables available and may also be loaded with sodium.

- If you have a week's worth of prepackaged meals in the house can you hold off eating everything at once? What about your family - will they sneak your meals and snacks when your back is turned?

You might also want to consider how much of a help it would be for you to learn to control your eating overall, and to learn how to cook so that you don't need to rely on packaged meals and restaurants.

Remember, Hoodia will help you to control your appetite for most of the day but it won't take it away completely. The decisions you make when you are hungry are going to greatly increase your chances of either losing the weight, staying where you are, or gaining more weight. You can't eat thousands of calories every day and then expect a simple pill to melt the fat off. So learning how to cook, how to sneak in some healthy options, and how to plan for your meals is going to help Hoodia do the job it needs to do all the more efficiently. Give these things some thought as they will mean not just weight loss but being healthier overall as well.

Five Important Steps to Putting it All Together

So how do we put this all together? How can you use Hoodia to help you with weight loss and with appetite suppressant? And how can you be sure that you're doing everything possible to let Hoodia help you?

Let's go over the steps needed to lose the weight you have, keep it under control, and use Hoodia properly so that you can get the best out of it.

STEP #1 - MAKE A PLAN.

You need to plan your eating and plan your physical activity, as well as remembering to take your Hoodia every day. Let's discuss how to do this.

Start with your eating. What are some good breakfast items, lunch items, and dinner menus you can come up with? Think of your schedule - breakfast may need to eaten quickly while you get yourself and the family out the door. If so you'll need a good low-sugar cereal or some granola you can eat on the run. It's time to start checking labels on those cereal boxes!

Lunch will mean something other than fast food, so you'll need to think about soup, sandwiches, and things such as these. What will you need for the entire week?

Plan all these things out for your dinner and snack items as well. Think of what will make a healthy dinner; check recipes if you need to brush up on your cooking. It also helps to write out on a calendar what you'll be eating for every single day. This way you won't eat all your foods at once and won't be wondering what's for dinner tonight! The more organized you are about your eating, the more in control you're going to be with your weight.

Your menu plan will mean a good shopping list. Make sure that you check your pantry to see what you already have on hand so you don't purchase too much.

Exercising and physical activity may also require a plan. You should treat it as you would any other important responsibility - put it on the calendar and commit yourself to it. Remember to start slow and easy and work your way up to something more strenuous. And rather than seeing when you have time on your calendar, *make* time for exercise. Think of what you can give up, whether it's your weekly poker game or playing video games two or three nights per week.

Your planning stage is where you also get the kids involved and ask for help from whomever might help you. Talk to a friend about joining an exercise class together or about getting together for yoga and aerobics on a regular basis. Investigate what options you have at home, whether it's buying some DVDs or looking through your cable's "on demand" options.

STEP #2 - START SMALL.

Remember that you probably took a long time to gain all the weight you're carrying so it will probably take some time for you to lose it as well. If you start too strenuously you may injure yourself and may also get discouraged very easily. So start small and make minor changes but keep them consistent. For exercise, start with walking for twenty minutes four or five times every week and then gradually increase that. Lift very light weights, just a few pounds worth. Switch up your exercising with other activities that you're doing with the family and with friends or your partner. Think about how you can make it fun but don't push yourself too hard all at once.

This means with your eating plan as well. You might find yourself craving your favorite foods as you make changes; trying to lose weight doesn't mean denying yourself completely. Just cut back or cut down - have fast food once per week rather than every day for lunch. Adjust to a smaller size meal. If you must have chocolate, have a bite-size portion rather than a full candy bar. Have light beer rather than regular when you do want a brew.

Substituting healthier food options is also going to make it easier for you to stick with this. You don't need to deny yourself a snack before bed but you should make it a piece of fruit or some low-fat microwave popcorn. Steam vegetables for side dishes for every meal so that you can fill up on them rather than the main course. Try wheat bread rather than white and do the same for pasta - most supermarkets now carry whole wheat pasta and other healthier options.

STEP #3 - MAKE PROGRESS.

Just because you need to start small doesn't mean that you should never challenge yourself or make some progress. Continue to reduce your portion sizes until you're eating the number of calories that are healthy for you every single day. Increase your physical activity and exercise until you can do this on a consistent basis without a problem. Add some resistance training to your workout and gradually increase how much you lift, staying within safe limits of course.

Challenging yourself is an important part of making progress. Some people become very complacent and even downright bored with their new routine but if you can change up what you do and how much, this will keep things fresh and new for you and can help stave off boredom.

And the more progress you make, the more weight you'll lose. If you don't challenge yourself and don't make progress your weight will eventually level off and you'll stop losing, and may even gain some of it back. So start small and stay manageable but continue to improve in both your eating and your exercise.

A good way to do this is to keep track of your eating and your physical activity. Note the progress you make on a calendar and note when you should be increasing your efforts as well. Tell yourself that starting next week you'll increase your walking by ten minutes each time or will try a different aerobic routine. Once you start going without fast food meals you may realize that you can go an entire week without hitting the drive-through, and a week turns into a month and so on.

When you keep track of what you're doing it's that much easier to challenge yourself and to be sure that you're making progress with both eating and exercise.

STEP #4 - TAKE YOUR HOODIA!

Hoodia is going to help you keep your eating under control even on your worst days and when you have your worst cravings. Many people are enthused about a new eating plan - for about a week. And then of course they return to their old habits and find themselves again eating out of boredom, frustration, to relieve tension and stress, or for reasons other than true hunger.

And this is where Hoodia can really help. As you try to gradually learn new habits, you won't be distracted with those hunger pangs that aren't really hunger pangs. You can go through your day without being obsessed with your next meal or your next snack.

Imagine how much weight you can lose and how you can get your weight under control if you no longer had those cravings before bedtime or could walk away from the dinner table after a modest meal. Your exercising would be more effective and your meals would be more satisfying and fulfilling overall.

Taking Hoodia is not some magic cure for obesity but is a very powerful weapon in the arsenal you need in your own battle of the bulge. And don't you want to use every weapon imaginable when it comes to weight loss?

Remind yourself of the benefits of Hoodia as well:

- All the clinical trials that have involved Hoodia have shown great results, with participants eating sometimes just half of what they were eating previously.

- So far there have been no reported side effects of Hoodia other than possible dehydration because of one's lack of thirst. Make sure you keep yourself hydrated while using it.

- If your appetite is under control you're more likely to lose weight, even if it means eating a hundred or so calories less than what you've been used to eating.

So don't ignore the use of Hoodia as well as all these other tips we've outlined. Every single thing you do to control your eating and to stay active is going to help to keep your weight under control.

STEP #5 - KEEP IT UP FOR LIFE!

There's probably nothing in the world more frustrating than losing weight only to gain it back, along with additional weight on top of that. So be prepared to keep up your new routine for life. Remind yourself of how good you feel when you lose weight and how much you hate it when you gain it back. This too is why you need to find exercise and physical activity you enjoy and should learn how to prepare food that is tasty. This can make it easier for you to stay with your new choices for life.

It also helps to consider why it is that you personally want to control your weight. Go back to the first section and reread all the ways obesity and excessive body weight affect your health. Take a moment to highlight or note the reasons that are personal to you. Maybe you have a history of heart problems in the family or are already starting to notice problems with your joints that will no doubt one day lead to arthritis. Or maybe your back is in near constant pain already. Or you and your partner are trying to get pregnant and didn't realize that obesity can cause problems with infertility for both men and women.

Think of your own reasons for wanting to stay healthy and in shape and make a note of them. Keep this list handy so that when you're ready to give up, you are reminded of why you should keep going. Take a look at your kids and think about what type of example you're setting for them and what habits you're teaching them. Ask yourself if you want them to learn unhealthy habits that will follow them for their life.

Hoodia can do a lot to keep your appetite in line so that you can learn how to cook and prepare your own meals and can also learn about healthy portion sizes. You can also exercise more often, as this gets easier as you lose more weight.

You owe it to yourself to keep up your good habits and to keep them up for life. So don't give up in your own battle of the bulge. It can be won, if you're determined to win and if you allow Hoodia to help!